Back Maintenance
&
Body Management

Back Maintenance & Body Management

A Unique Method

Developed by

Raul E. Nava

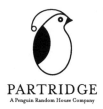

PARTRIDGE

A Penguin Random House Company

ISBN: Softcover   978-1-4828-3254-9
            eBook   978-1-4828-3255-6

Print information available on the last page.

To order additional copies of this book, contact
Toll Free 800 101 2657 (Singapore)
Toll Free 1 800 81 7340 (Malaysia)
orders.singapore@partridgepublishing.com

www.partridgepublishing.com/singapore

Contents

Preface

I was a little more than eight years old when my Lola Iska called me aside into her little room to say that I should be taking her instructions a little bit more seriously because she's not always available to give my mother the treatment for her migraine attacks. She expected me to start giving my mother the treatment in her place. 'I'll try…' I just said. Even at that young age I was one who would never back out from a challenge.

Lola Iska was not our real grandmother. She came as a household help just before I was born and as far back as I remember we considered her as our true grandmother. She came from a very small and remote barrio and from a family of 'arbolarios' or healers. And although she knew all the herbal treatments, the oil massages, the manipulations and incantations – she could never become the 'accepted' healer because that passed from father to son. She was the younger of two sisters. So, with a heavy heart she went to the town and to work in our family. This did not stop her from giving treatments within the family circle. Even our neighbors would come for a variety of reasons and she would treat them.

From the beginning, I was fascinated by the healing techniques that she used and would often ask questions – a lot of questions. She never lost patience with me. Instead, she would meticulously describe each anomaly, questions to ask the patient, how to look for telltale signs of skin color and texture, eyes, posture, timbre of the voice, and many more. She showed me how to use the oils and the herbs, let me feel the right pressure of manipulation, to arouse the tones of muscles and organs, to lower fever and rejuvenate body forces, and many, many more. In the end, I must have been a good learner because after a while my mother would call only for me. At about the same time I developed my own variation to treat my mother's migraine attacks so that in a very short while she would become fast asleep (even lightly snoring). And soon, I was off with my friends to play outside. She would later complain about my abandoning her. And I would simply say: 'If you were fast asleep by the time I left, it means that you were feeling all right…so, I left!'

I come from a family of physicians. My father was a Pediatrician, several cousins and several uncles are all surgeons. And so, I was expected to study Medicine as well. But I refused to become a physician. Maybe the deep rooted reason behind my refusal has something to do with the hardship my father underwent as I accompanied him at times – late at night, in the middle of heavy rain, when he would come back to the car where he had left me behind to watch – angry and cursing because he fell into a wet rice patch when he missed a turn. Sometimes he would come back after a very long time with a bound chicken and a handful of vegetables because that was what the family could afford to pay.

My 'mea culpa' was that in the long run, I turned a full circle and am now deeply involved in the art of healing – be it in the form of the other kind: Complementary Medicine.

In the late 1980's I convinced my kibbutz to send me to China for advanced studies in Chinese Medicine and to concentrate on Tuina after I got a very warm recommendation from Dr. Hua Dong who was in charge of our Tuina course.

He complemented my technique and was thoroughly surprised to find out that I learned it from my Lola Iska. I set out for a half year program of advanced learning and 'internship' at Jinan, in the province of Shandong – China.

We started off as a group of 15 Israelis studying at two levels, staying together at the University of Shandong's Foreign Students' dormitory and doing our work at the University hospital. After 12 weeks all have left except me. I asked the University for a special, advanced program in Tuina and Acupuncture. It was granted and Dr. Guan Zheng at the Tuina Department of the University Hospital took me under his personal care. It was during this intensive daily routine that my knowledge broadened, deepened, and literally matured.

As I started my work as a regular member of Dr. Guan Zheng's staff, I was given to treat an elderly woman who was suffering from chronic, severe back pains. She has been coming regularly and enduring the hard handed and really painful treatments and manipulations. Oftentimes the patients would groan out loud and sometimes even shed a tear or two. I started to give her my treatment – Tuina with more than the usual and normal energetic technique that I give to my patients. As I was going through the leg and hip manipulation, she let out a cry that startled the whole section. "Hey, Professor!" she shouted. "This young one over here (referring to me) – he's not hurting me! But it's easing the pain – just as effectively!!!" Dr. Guan Zheng just looked at her, smiled knowingly and quite laconically said: "Ah, yes – that's Israeli style!!!" (It didn't even occur to them that I'm Filipino!)

As I developed the 'Israeli' style of treatment, more and more people- old and younger ones alike, have come to enjoy the benefits that this unique technique has to offer. It was not long before I developed the system of Back Maintenance and Body Management – a unique set of exercises to help us keep fit. Its main aim is to attain a healthy mind and an equally healthy body.

Introduction

It has been said that from the time man saw the benefits derived by walking on his hind legs aside, of course, with a few minor drawbacks – he has always paid his dues and dividends – in the form of various forms of back pains. And he had to find ways with which to find relief for them. The first way – and he almost had no choice about it - was physical labor. And as a matter of fact, too hard and too much of it added more to his woes. A good days' manual labor in fact strengthened his back. He kept himself in good shape.

But man went on from physical labor to utilizing machines to do his work. The use of machines and of push buttons gradually saw him using less and less of his body and he began to grow weaker and back pains became an even more severe problem.

The 1970's and 80's saw an upsurge of interest in various forms of exercises- mainly jogging, walking, aerobics, and with the gradual acceptance of the Alternative Medicine which later came to be generally accepted as Complementary Medicine since it looked upon itself as a partner of Western Medicine – other various forms of exercises were introduced such as Yoga, Self-Shiatsu, Self-Tuina, Tai Chi, Chi Kung, as well as the lesser known ones that were developed such as Pilatis, Feldenkriez, the Paula Technique – to mention but a few. The more vigorous forms were favored by the young. And though these exercises increased their muscles they did not seem to help relieve the back pains. On the contrary, not a few cases worsened by the heavy impact caused by exertive running and hard aerobics. Also, there were some bad effects brought about by even the simplest form of walking just by the reaction of the body – the back, specifically, simply because it wasn't done right. The older people rightly chose to do the less rigorous forms and done right – benefited them a lot.

There are several reasons why we experience back problems from simple back aches to the chronically more irritable pains.

The first main reason may lie in the fact that we were born with the problem or rather, we inherited the problem in our genes which we have very little to do except to correct it by surgery and a lot of physiotherapy treatment and exercises.

Another reason may be from injuries we may have sustained for many reasons or through our own fault by wrong actions of lifting, pulling or pushing very heavy objects.

Other reasons come from our daily work routine such as sitting for long hours without taking time to stretch and relax a little bit. Within the same context may be repetitive work that involves the same set of muscular movement during the whole eight hour shift. Blowers, fans, air conditioners or heaters all affect our body and contribute to aggravate back pains.

There is however, a very important yet almost always overlooked factor that contribute to all those pains that we feel. In fact, we even tend to disregard it altogether and accept it as part of our daily lives. I refer to that little part in ourselves that make up all that we sense and feel.

In my many years of practicing Complementary Medicine I have come to realize that our mental well being and balance contribute a lot not only to the healing process within us but prevents a loot of abnormalities that could occur by those imbalances.

We live and work in an atmosphere that is filled with a lot of tension and pressure – pressure to achieve goals that are set by ourselves or by others; pressure of deadlines to finish a given task or to attain maximum profit in business endeavors; pressure to be able to be faster, bigger, higher – to be the best!

All these come with a price – too much strain on our minds, feelings, senses that affect not only our interpersonal relations but more importantly - our own health.. Too much irritability, anger, worry, fear, sadness, and yes – even too much joy could greatly affect our health. In Chinese Medicine, a certain feeling is attributed to a specific organ of our body. The principle states that joy balances sadness; anger balances calmness; etc.

Keeping this body-sense equation in mind, we can thus come to the conclusion that in order to have a healthy body we must avoid too strong emotions in our daily life. Great thinking ! – but almost too impossible to achieve! Just try forgetting a long kept hate you've harbored for a long time inside – within your heart!

Complementary Medicine gives us tools for us to deal with this aspect. We can do Yoga, meditation exercises – transcendental and other meditative forms, relaxation techniques, as well as Reiki, Healing Hands, and Harmonious Body/ Mind exercises.

A body that is in disharmony with the Mind/ Spirit is liable to feel the effect in various ways – more importantly – pain in various parts of the body. Back pains – from the lower part to the upper back as well as the neck, the arms and the legs are just a few of what we feel.

And this being so, I have come to a very simple yet startling conclusion which I have come to develop throughout the years by the various classes and patients I have taught and cared for. I call this concept – ***The Principle of Body Management and Back Maintenance***

Head, Neck and Upper Body Warm-up

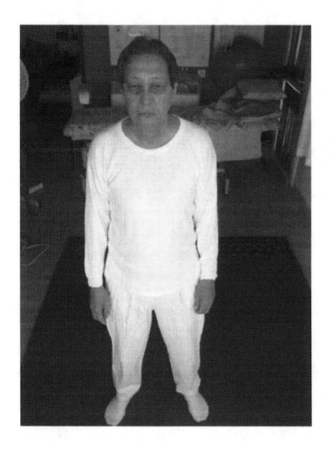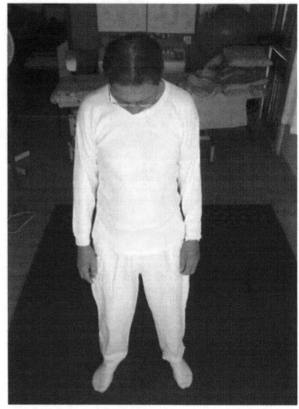

Lower your head till the chin is touching the upper part of the breast. Try to be aware of bending each vertebra of the neck from the Atlas to C-7 exhaling slowly as you do so; keep your head down for three regular breaths and to straighten the head once more – just as slowly- inhaling as you do.

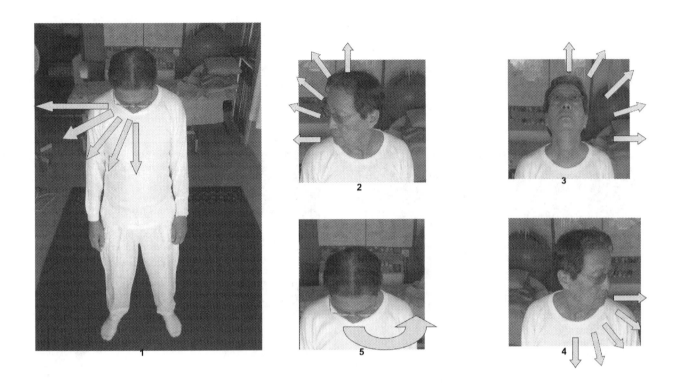

Revolve your head first by again bringing the head down till the chin rests upon the upper breast; moving to the right side along the floor not in one motion but dividing your movement in such a way as you move you head to three distinct points along the right side of the floor, three points along the right wall from the bottom up, divide the ceiling into six points, another three points along the left wall, and finally – three points along the left floor till the head is again straight down. Do the same but towards the left side first until done. Repeat the exercise three times. Dividing the head's rotation along these points help to prevent feeling dizzy. Also, refrain from tilting your head too far backward.

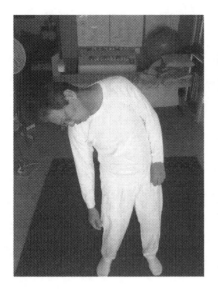 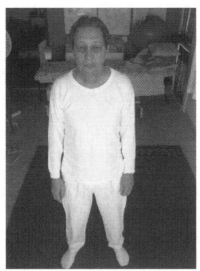 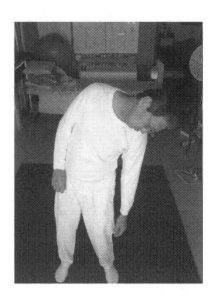

Inhale deeply and upon exhaling gently, slowly bend your upper body down to your left side followed by your head as if you want to touch the tip of your shoulder with your left ear. Straighten back up slowly, inhaling as you do. Do the same thing towards the right side. Repeat the exercise tree times.

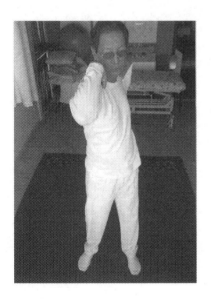 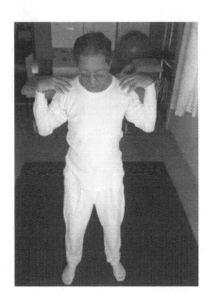 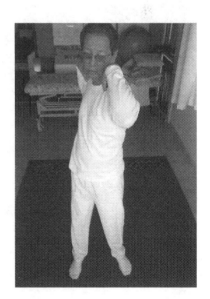

Touch both tips of your shoulders with your fingertips lightly and start to rotate your elbows – first the left and then the right – in a forward motion for three times and then backwards for another three times.

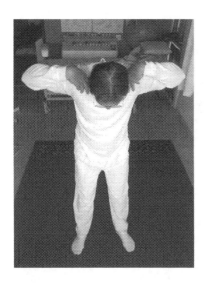 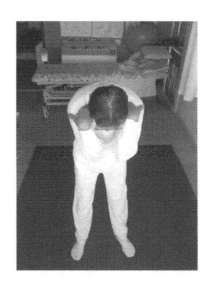 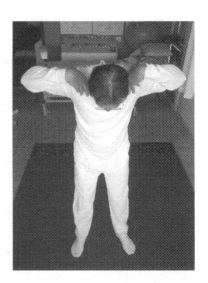

Still with the fingers upon your shoulder tips, make as though you are flapping wings but with your elbows instead. Do this movement also three times.

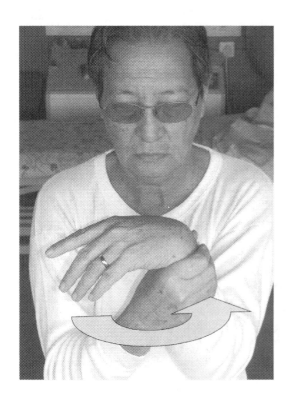 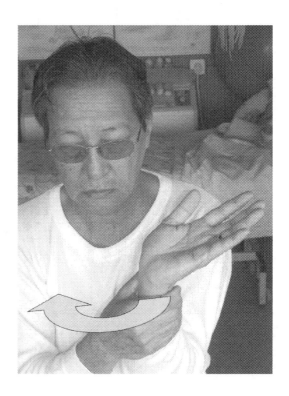

Wrap the fingers of your right hand around the left wrist lightly – for support- and slowly rotate the left hand three times towards the left and another three times towards the right.

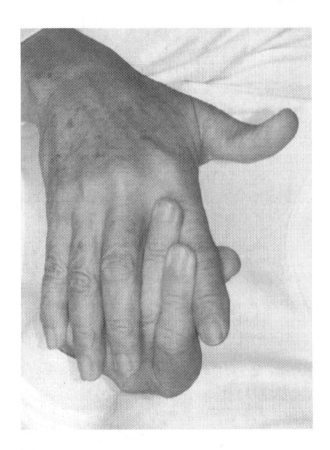 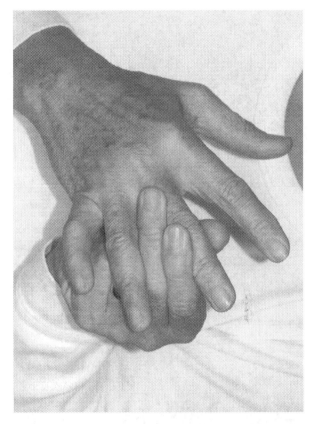

Gently massage each joint of each finger of the hand in a circular motion for several seconds with the other hand. Repeat massage on the other hand.

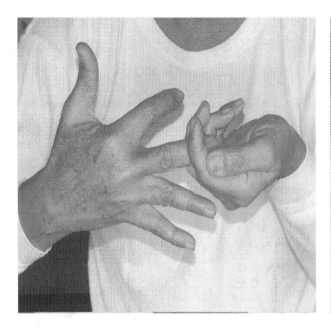
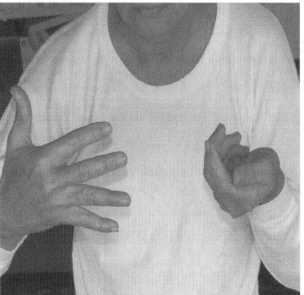

Now, gently but firmly hold each finger with the forefinger and ring finger of the other hand and with the same pressure swiftly release the finger. Producing a snapping sound takes a bit of practice. It is believed that this action enhances the flow of the upper body's Yin-Yang energies.

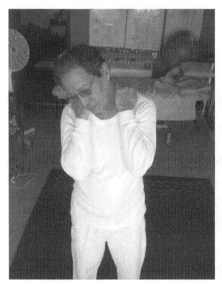
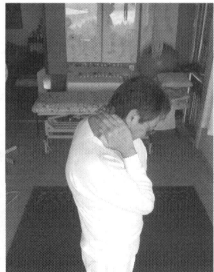
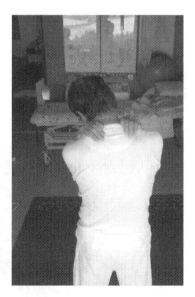

Gently grasp and massage the area around the nape and the top area of each shoulder while slowly swaying the head from side to side.

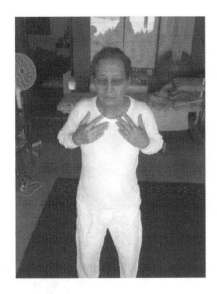
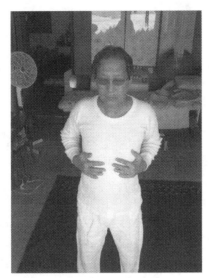
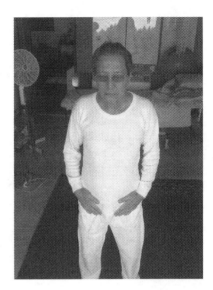

Softly rub both the front part and the sides of your ribs with both hands —
checking for knotted muscles and loosening them up.

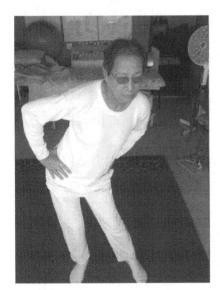
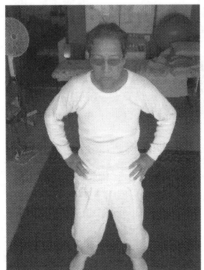
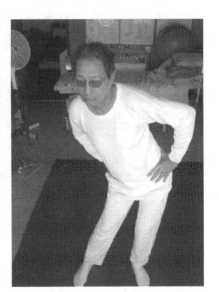

With hands on your hips gently gyrate clockwise as well as counter-clockwise
for a couple of seconds. Take special care to move only the mid-portion of the
body.

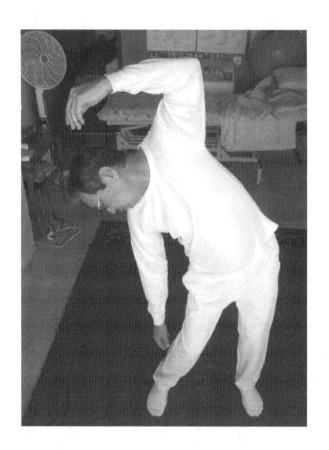 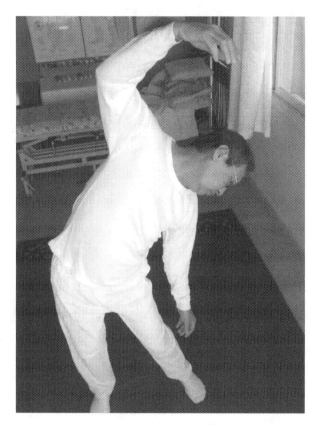

Standing straight with legs a bit apart, bend the body from the hips towards the left and raise the hand at the same time. Do the same towards the right. Inhale before each bending and exhale slowly as you bend. Do this three times on each side.

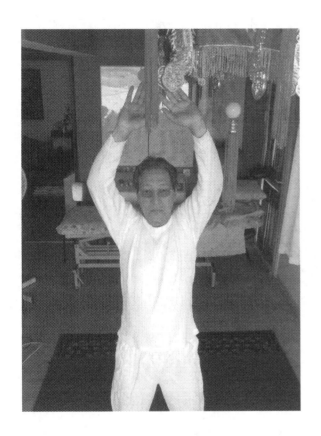 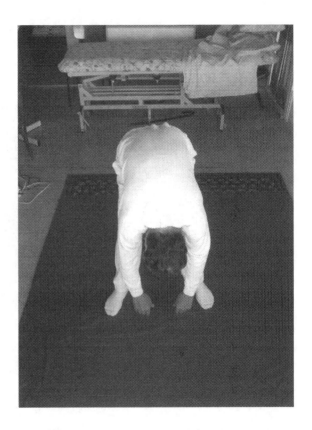

Raise both hands, inhale deeply and as you exhale bend down from the lower back part of the hips as far as you can comfortably go down. Don't straighten nor lock the knees – they impair the movement and cramp the muscles. Try to feel the opening up of each vertebra from the sacrum to the neck bones. After a couple of short breaths while you are bent down – slowly inhale and straighten up the body again from the sacrum up to the neck and head.

Lower body parts –Warm up

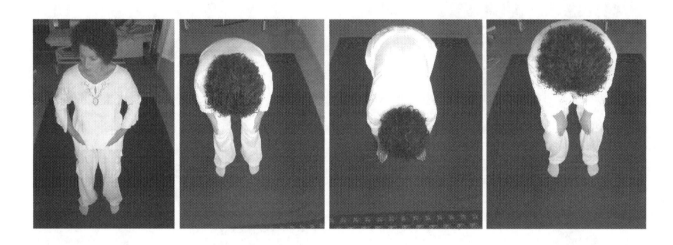

Bring your hands towards both sides of the groin and with slow breathing, rub both sides of your outer legs from the hips down to the tips of our feet, rounding about the toes and then straightening up still rubbing the legs but this time the inner part till you come to a stop again at the groins. The exercise is made a lot easier if you don't lock your knees.

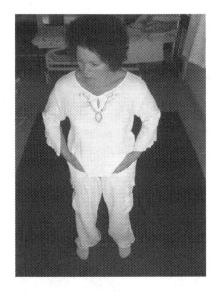
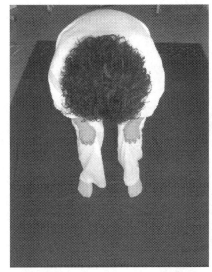
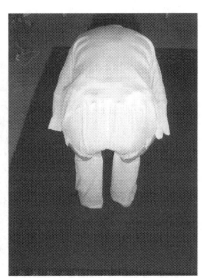

Repeat the same up and down movement while lightly rubbing your legs but instead of going all the way down, stop at the knees and gently massage both the front and back part of the knees. (X3)

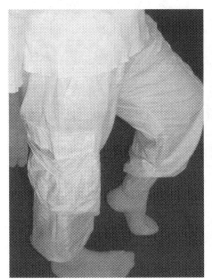
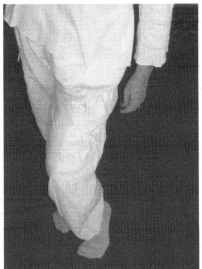
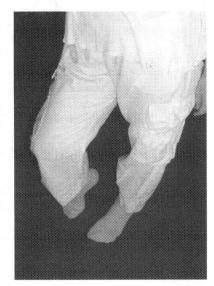

In this exercise, move like you're climbing up the stairs but don't lift your feet – only the soles and the toes go up and down and make greater use of your hips –although a little bit exaggerated…(repeat 3 times)

Sitting Down Exercises

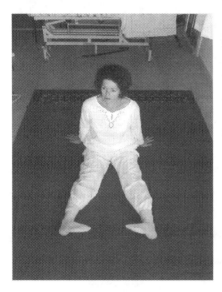 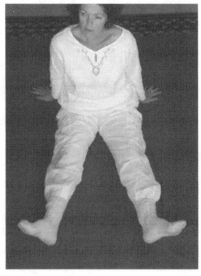 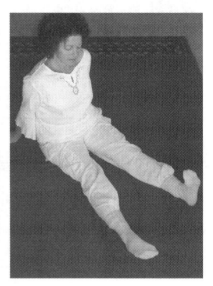

Sitting down with your legs a bit apart and straight start to rotate your foot together first in one direction and then the other for not more than three times and continue to bend them forward and back – much like you were stepping on the gas and on the brakes with one foot then the other (also 3X)

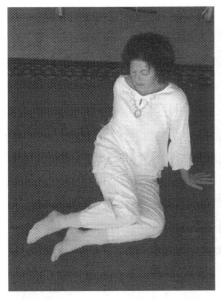 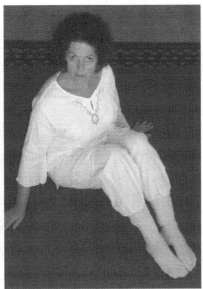 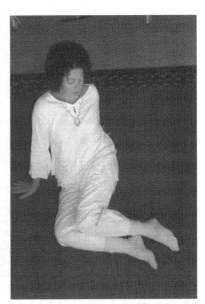

Now bring up your knees together and with your arms firmly on your sides move them from side to side making certain that you open up the muscles of hips and waist area.

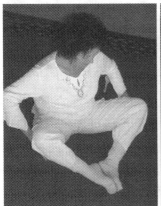 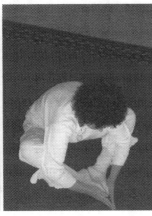 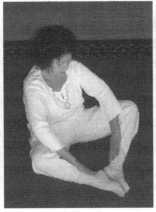 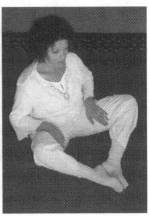

Still sitting down, bring your soles together opening and bringing down your knees to as much as we comfortably can. After a brief moment of getting used to, start the rubbing exercise of the outer part of your legs down to the toes and the upward movement from the toes back to the groin along the inner part of the legs. Make a bobbing motion as you do this exercise making certain that you exhale as you bend down and inhale as you straighten up. (3X)

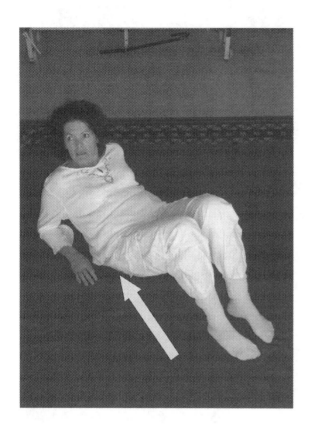 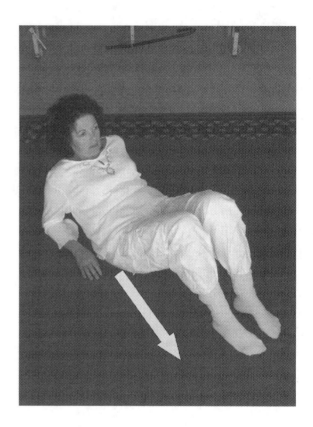

Assume the position - halfway between sitting and lying down knees bent upwards Start to undulate forward and backward while all the time feeling that you're opening up your lower back from the sacrum towards the whole length of the lumbar vertebrae and even further if you slightly lift your tailbone (coccyx).

Use your elbows for support on this particular exercise.

Back Maintenance Exercises

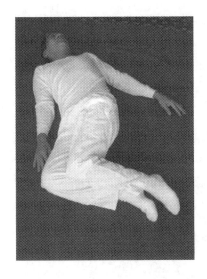 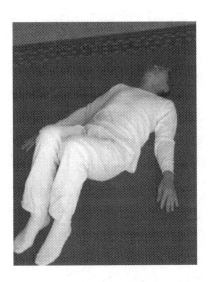 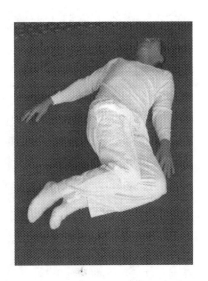

Lying upon your back, bring your knees upward and together. Move them from side to side just as you did sitting down – only, this time you feel less resistance upon your movements. Keep your shoulders flat, all your movements for the following exercises require only your hips and the lower portion of your body. As always: do this three times – no more.

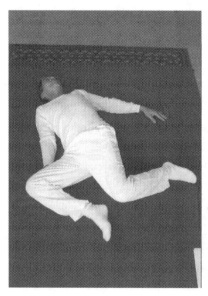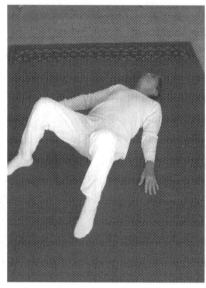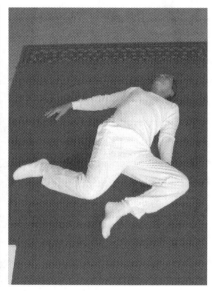

Repeat the same exercise but with the legs and knees spread apart. Notice that by moving the left knee downward followed by the right – you are lifting the side of your hips higher that the previous exercise. This allows a gradual opening up of the vertebrae along the lower back area. (3X)

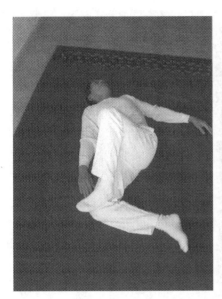 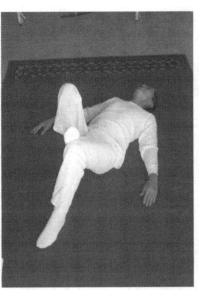 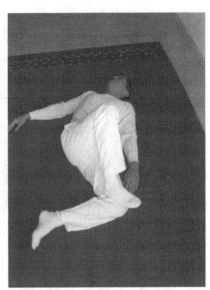

Now place the right foot over the left knee and slowly move the left leg from side

to side. The distance from the floor depends on how comfortable you can bring

it down. After three repetitions, change the upright leg to the right and complete

the same exercise. Notice that you bring up the side of your hips to its greatest

angle thus opening the spines of your lower back to the utmost.

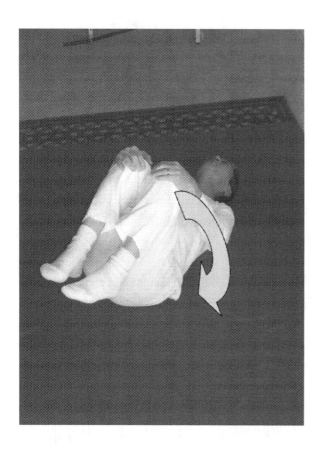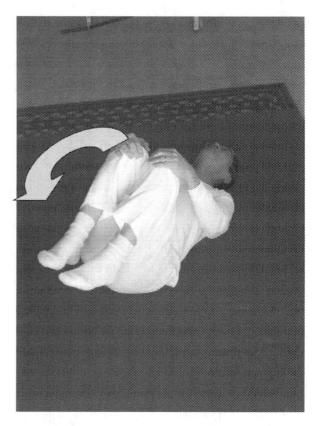

Resume supine position holding your knees upwards. Gently rock your whole body from side to side with the movement being centered upon your lower back.

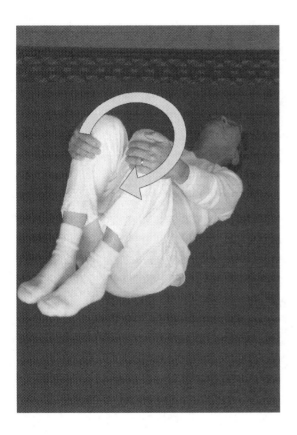 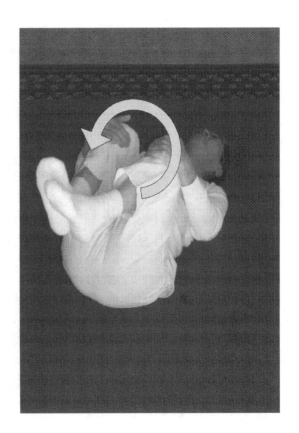

After a couple of seconds rotate your knees in a circular motion first towards one direction and then towards the other.

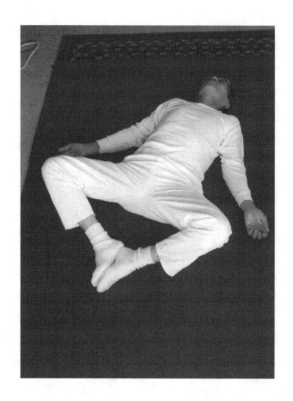

Place the soles of your foot together and gently let the knees and the legs open sideward. Feel the gradual loosening of the thigh muscles and the opening up of the groin areas. (Again, 3X)

Exercises On All Fours

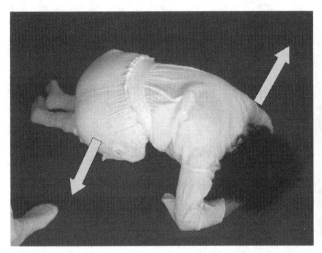 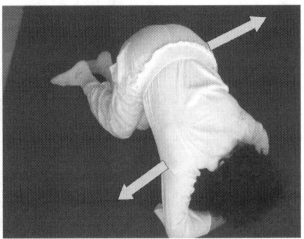

Turn over on all fours – a crouching position – with both your hands under your forehead. Start by rocking yourself with the movement emanating both from the lower back as well as the shoulders. This will gradually loosen the entire length of the back muscles.

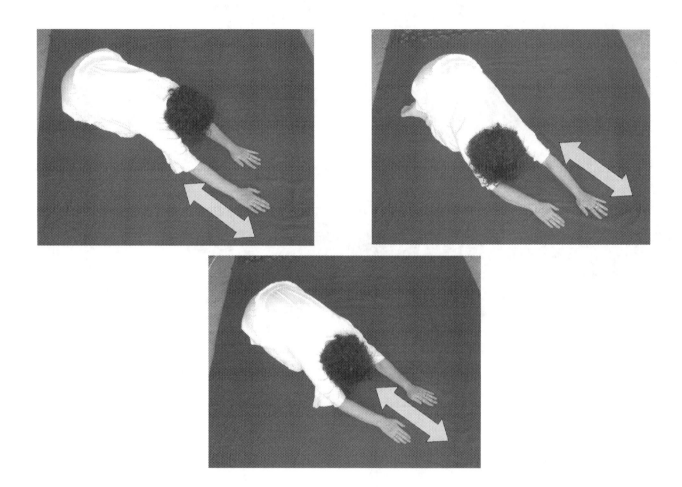

You then extend your arms forward and start to reach out- one hand after the other (3 times) and finally stretch out with both hands as far as you comfortably can.

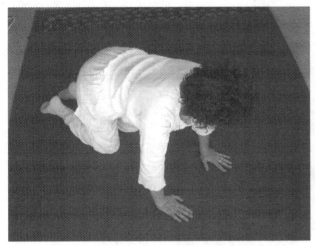 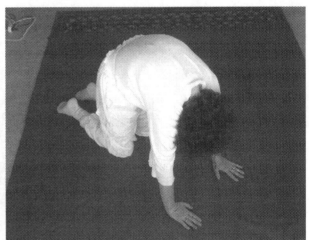

Return to your crouching position; slowly and gently arch your back upward and then straighten back - take care not to arch them down so as not to put extra strain on the spine –(3 times, no more).

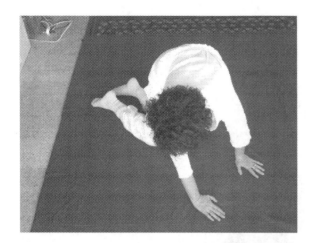 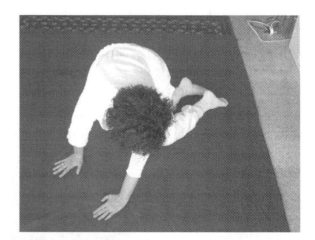

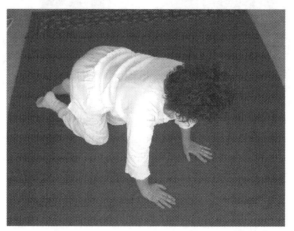

You then proceed to turn your body from the left side then the right side as if to look at the soles of your feet.

Upper Body Exercises

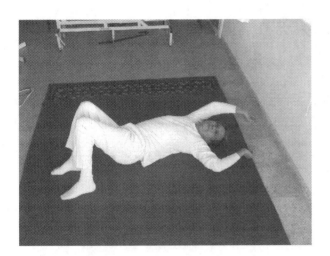 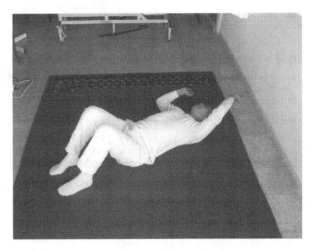

Lie down upon your back, gently position your arms over your head and stretch one hand after the other as though you are stretch-yawning.

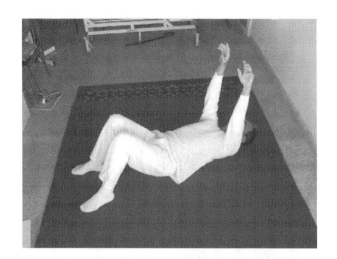

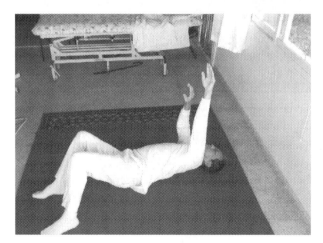
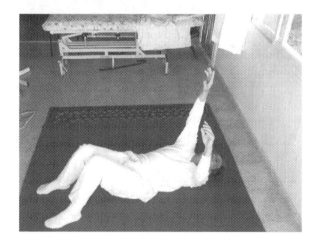

Still lying upon your back with both arms up toward the ceiling, lift an arm together with the shoulder as if you want to touch the ceiling. Three times, then proceed to lift the other arm. The exercise is made easier with your knees also bent upwards.

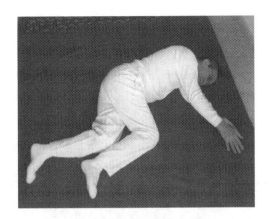

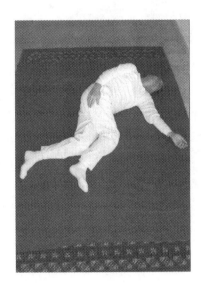
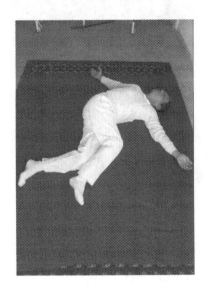
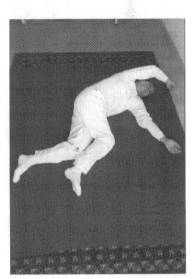

Lie sidewards with both hands forward – left leg straight behind the right leg which is slightly bent. Then rotate your arm in a 'lazy' manner three times in one direction and then another three times in the other. Then turn over to the other side and do the same exercise with the other arm

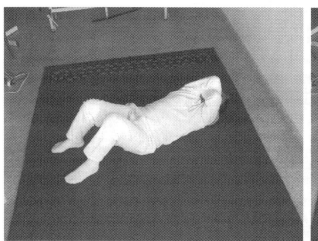 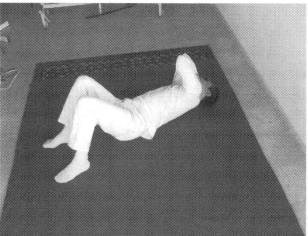

Lastly, embrace your shoulders and sway from side to side as though you're lulling yourself to relaxation.

Combination Exercises

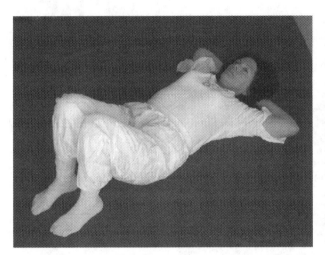 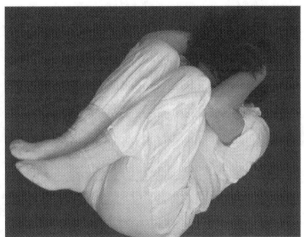

Start by lying supine on your back – knees bent upwards and your hands supporting the back of your head. With each exhalation bring the head and the knees as closely together as deliberately and comfortably possible. Return to the supine position at the start of inhaling as slowly and as deliberately as at the start of the movement – try not to jerk the body...

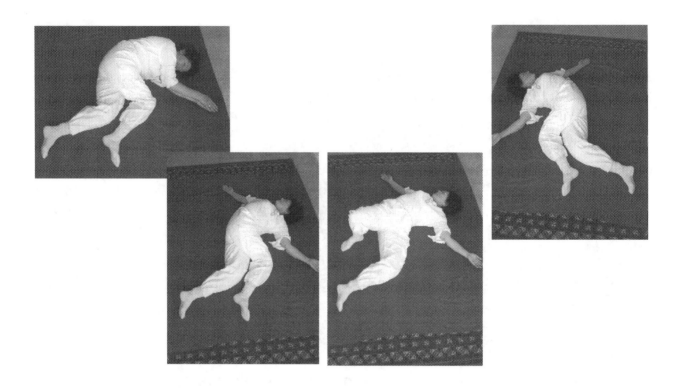

Next, lie on your side with both arms lightly extended and one leg over the other slightly bent. Almost in a 'lazy' manner move an arm over to the other side- relax for about a breath's time- follow with the leg and without hurrying – the other leg and finally the second arm that has up to this point remained in place. This is called the – Arm-Leg-Leg-Arm exercise. Try not to overexert yourself.

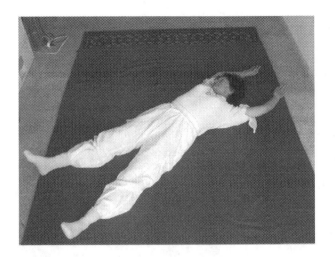
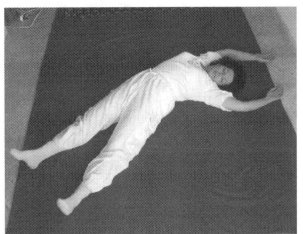

Lie on your back with your legs straight and spread them a little bit. Your arms are once again extended over your head. Reach with a slight stretch up with you left arm and shoulder and at the same time move your left hip and leg downwards in a bending-elongating motion. Do the same on the right side.

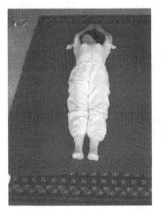
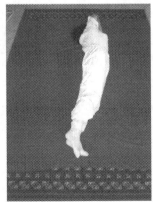
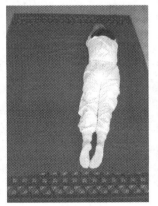
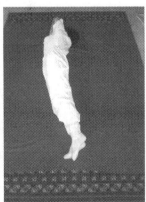

Still with your arms extended over your head – gently roll to the right side upon your stomach – roll back up supine – and then roll back to your stomach but toward the left side. This is a very exhilarating exercise. You can do this exercise more than three times.!!!

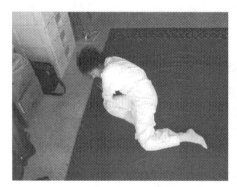 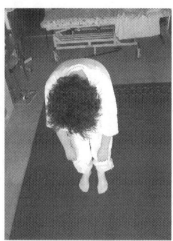 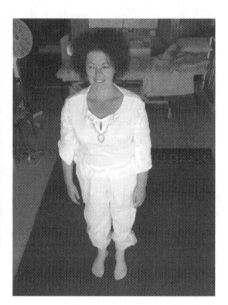

Slowly stand up and with a relaxed stance, assume the position we had at the start of the very first exercise.

Conclusion And Recommendations

As we grow older, the effects of years upon years of work, daily routine, exercises (mostly strenuous and prolonged), heavy lifting, pushing, pulling – are all gradually felt and are added to our continually growing list of aches and pains. Even if we reduce the strain and the tension in our way of living, ours is a one way path progressing towards the inevitable end.

The <u>Principles of Body Maintenance – Back Management</u> does not claim to heal chronic pains and maladies mainly because of the complexity of problems involving such pains. Problems of Osteoporosis, atrophy of both muscles and bones, changes in bone structures, etc., are but some of the reasons that contribute to such complexities. The body also has such a dynamic nature that a lot of changes occur as time passes. However, we do know one thing: we can ease the acute pains; we have a solution to those nagging back aches. Even if the pains do not permanently go away, we can always do the exercises to greatly relieve ourselves even for a while. It is very encouraging to hear from a couple of members of a country club where I give lessons in Back Maintenance claiming how miserable they felt before we started the lesson and how the pain simply went away as we progressed through the exercises.

These exercises were carefully selected and chosen through many years of giving treatments, actual lessons and workshops with the elderly utmost in our minds. But this does not mean that the younger people can't participate. On the contrary, I have been approached by a lot of youngsters, even teenagers wondering if I could recommend it to them. I gave them a lot of encouragement and advised them to join the group. They have not regretted the decision to exercise with us ever since. I even had a workshop for young would be mothers. Although they were in different degrees of pregnancy, everyone thoroughly enjoyed the lessons. Not only did they have normal and easy childbirth, I see their children – now walking and running about – all very active and in perfect health.

By its nature, the exercises are all done in a very relaxed way.

As I have stated, we refrain from taking meals before we exercise. We do not want our systems – especially the digestive system to work at the same time that we are doing our exercises.

And how often do we exercise?

I have suggested to my group – composed mainly of elderly people to know themselves a little better and to feel their own capabilities, to be aware of when the pains bother them most, to know what they did that gave way to pains, and to try to alleviate appropriately and comfortably. Also, one does not need to do all the exercises to maintain one's health. As time goes by, we will have developed a fond liking for some particular exercise and find ourselves going over that 'favorite' exercise again and again. The motto is: "If it makes you feel good – there's no way that can stop you from doing it."

This book is our first step towards the proper and natural way to a healthy and maintained body – less aches, less pains, and certainly, a lot more aware of the beauty, the love, and the joy of simple – LIVING!!!

Raul E. Nava

October 2007

This Book

*This book is a careful and loving compilation of many years worth of experience in different aspects of Complementary Medicine. Patients, as well as non-patients who have undergone treatments, seminars, workshops and special courses with me all contributed in their own special way to the development and building up of the various exercises.

*This book was written to serve as a guide and to give the reader a very basic but compact view of the various forms of movements in our attempt to solve back problems. There are countless variations. However, in no way should we regard the contents of this book as a medical remedy or professional health guide to general or specific maladies. Utmost care should be taken while doing the exercises. The author and publisher will not take liability nor responsibility to anyone with regards to any injury or physical damage caused or alleged to be caused directly or indirectly by the information contained in this book.

*This book would probably have not seen light without the constant support and encouragement by my wife, Racheli, who was always there to give some words of comfort and help. Heartfelt thanks, also, to Dani Hyman for diligently translating together with Lea Tessler, and for patiently photographing the whole series; to Hind for her fabulous meals making us feel always at home even though away from home,,, and finally, to all my family:

my daughter and my son, and my sisters;

my friends, pupils, acquaintances, and everyone who took such deep interest and understanding from the time they heard that an idea of a book is about to be – born...

He is the wise one – to whom the beginning and the end is clear"

Confucius

Unique methods of healing were developed by unique people...

Raul E. Nava was born to a pediatrician and was brought up by a nanny who was well trained in the art of the unconventional healing methods of treatment. So, the little child grew up and was exposed to this atmosphere. His soul and body filled with this unconventional practice and knowledge at a very young age.

At eight (8) years old he was helping his nanny give treatments to his mother's bouts of migraine and severe headaches.

Two years as a medical student made him realize that his future is not to follow in the footsteps of his father but to go along the path of his beloved nanny.

After long studies and half a year of advanced learning and working in China he began to sow the seeds of healing and care, giving hope to hundreds of patients and pupils that he taught and treated. As he gained experience and depth of knowledge, he began to compile and organize them into a unique method – a system that he called:

BACK MAINTENANCE and BODY MANAGEMENT

This book is a revolution if you compare it to all the known methods of self treatment in the care of all forms of back pains. It is simple, well created and easy to perform, so that anyone of all ages and from all walks of life can practice. Most important, it can be done at group meetings and social happenings once or twice a week.

This little book is a must in our daily way of life and should have an important place on every family's bookshelf.